SEXYFITYOU

Guide to SexyFitYou Lifestyle

CLARA CHIZOBA KRONBORG

AuthorHouse™ UK
1663 Liberty Drive
Bloomington, IN 47403 USA
www.authorhouse.co.uk
Phone: 0800.197.4150

Published by AuthorHouse 02/26/2019

ISBN: 978-1-7283-8526-6 (sc)
ISBN: 978-1-7283-8525-9 (e)

author**HOUSE**®

Now let me introduce to you SexyFitYou. ☺

Contents

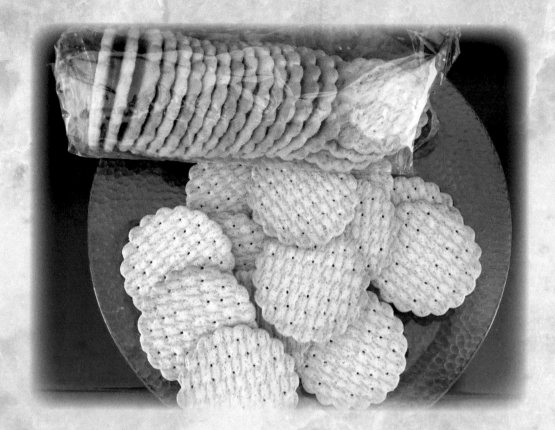

Yes , I have a weakness too , maybe just like you do. Mine is a biscuit—and a particular brand! So get comfortable and be guilt-free as I share with you how I built the SexyFitMe lifestyle.

Introduction

Recently, there has been so much awareness on women's need to love the shape and size they are. I'm a big fan of the idea because that reduces the pressure that the modern social media world causes us. But what worries me most is when others take advantage of this campaign and eat unnecessarily unhealthy because they believe they're fat because they were "created that way." Health-wise, no, but you should know that the sizes we are in, in most cases, are our choices.

SexyFitYou is one of my numerous ventures. But unlike other more recent things I do, I have been asking questions about fitness and health since I was a child, trying to find out how to live differently from the society I was surrounded by. Growing up, I had some family and friends who suffered so much from issues related to being overweight, such as diabetes, high blood pressure, and so on—not just a family member but my own dear mother.

When I was a child, we lived in a public yard (as we used to call it), where the stairs had no rail. It was only a two-floor building, but Mum had struggles climbing up and down the stairs. The worst of it was that she fell twice, with serious injuries at the time. Luckily she survived the falls and the injuries. She literally waited on each stair to catch her breath before she continued to climb. Before my mum died in 2017, I had the privilege to spend time with her as I never had before, and we talked virtually about everything. Among the topics was her wish that she'd never allowed herself to become fat. During her early years, and still in most places where I come from in Nigeria, Africa, a woman being fat was a symbol of wealth. She was seen as well taken care of by her husband, evidence of "good living", as they used to say.

My mum's sister had a Mercedes-Benz back then, and each time she and my mum got in it, the car literally went flat. No offence, Mum (may your soul rest on) and Aunty, I love you both. The fact was not that they were fat but that they were suffering from it. They had challenges getting out of bed, wearing clothes, and so on. I couldn't have been more motivated to live a different lifestyle, because I never wanted to go through what they'd gone through.

Adding to my motivation was watching most fat women being forced to pay for double seats in public transport; that included my mum too.

My environment motivated me. I wanted to live a different lifestyle and at a low cost.

Then it all started back when I left for boarding school in Enugu, Nigeria. I skipped dining time and gave out my food to school daughters (school daughter is a junior student that you choose to takecare of or simply said a junior student you mentor e.g follow ups in her academic performance etc) . ☺ I used to tell some of my friends then that I was doing 0-1-0, which is skipping breakfast and dinner, eating only lunch. Unhealthy, you might think now, but you haven't heard the worst of it. At fifteen years, I was drinking some slimming tea; I had zero idea of the damage it could have done to my body. That was how desperate I was to never be fat, but I was all going in the wrong direction. I realize that years later.

Fast forward to 2010 when I participated in one of my church organization's running event. That run changed my life. That was actually the first time I'd run (except for primary and secondary school PE activities). The run was only about two kilometres, but my body ached for days. Still, there was this feeling that I can't explain which kept my energy level unexpectedly high. I knew I wanted to try again, and I did. Again became again and again.

At first I would wake up at 5:00 a.m. because I had to leave for work at 7:00 a.m. and run about 2–3km, five days a week. And after each run, I would do my stretches, which I googled online how to do, and I did only twenty abs and twenty squats. I drank lots of water, and in less than one month, my body tone and energy level was at its peak. Then I thought, *Why not have a day rest from running after every two days?* I did. I noticed I had a quest to try new routes, new exercises, and to increase my running distance, but above all of this, I realized my eating habits had gotten better. I was basically eating everything I deprived myself of in boarding school.

Years went by, I became more friendly with my body, with every bite of food, every exercise and every change I felt. Is something you will see and feel when you get comfortable looking at yourself in the mirror and listening to only your needs. That is to say, be selfish when it comes to your needs,, your needs comes first. I wasn't a fat girl, but my quest was to maintain my desired shape and size.

Where I finally found myself, in terms of food was totally on *portion control* and *substituting*.

As you continue reading, you will find out how I place my thoughts at each level, and I hope you might pick one or two things that will help you maintain a SexyFitYou lifestyle.

Anyone who knows me knows how passionate I am about my fitness routines and, at the same time, how much I love a good, balanced meal.

Yes, I do love to snack between meals. And to top it all, I love a glass of good wine.

You might be wondering how I maintained being SexyFit. But the big questions are, What do I eat when I want to eat, and how often do I exercise?

Here is the thing about SexyFitYou. It is not a fitness, weight-loss, or muscle-building program. Rather, it is a lifestyle. You take your time to build yourself to the level where you are absolutely in control of your body. The SexyFitYou program encourages people, especially women, to be more active (exercise) and eat clean, not to bore themselves with dieting.

The word *sexy* takes some people's minds somewhere else, not that it's bad to spice up your thoughts. ☺ But here is the breakdown of the word *SexyFitYou*. It is about you loving yourself by feeling sexy in the shape you desire and being fit in that shape, while being yourself and not changing your personality in the process.

SexyFitYou is simply explained as the following:

Be sexy (self-love).

Be fit (active body and mind).

Be you (maintain your personality).

The Major Key Is Discipline

Just like everything else we do in life that requires discipline to succeed, SexyFitYou needs you to build up a discipline level which does not only require exercise and clean eating but also keeping a positive mindset that you can do it.

Building the discipline of being more active starts with our daily activities. For example, try the following:

- Instead of driving two kilometres, walk.
- Instead of using the elevator, climb the stairs.
- Children think it is fun to watch Mummy do lunges around the house. Try it; you will have an amazing time with your child.
- Dancing around while doing chores or playing with your kids at home is a good cardio exercise.

Clara's Weight-Maintaining Grocery List

Veggies

- leeks
- kale
- spinach
- cabbages
- broccoli
- carrots
- mushrooms
- grains
- okra
- cucumbers
- tomatoes
- pumpkin or pumpkin vegetable leaves

Proteins

- fish
- chicken
- beef
- turkey
- mussels
- shrimp

Fruits

- oranges
- apples
- bananas
- pineapples
- watermelon
- honeydew

Seasonings

- sea salt
- black pepper
- coconut oil/olive oil/pear oil
- garlic
- ginger
- curry
- basil leaves, dried
- mustard
- butter
- apple cider vinegar
- lemon

Daily

- eggs
- cheese
- milk (low-fat preferably)

Grains/Carbohydrates

- oatmeal
- whole wheat
- corn
- brown rice
- yams
- pastas (whole-grain pastas preferably)

Snacks

- almonds
- raisins
- coconut, dried

It is important to understand your body and its needs. Some persons have allergies or other reasons for not eating foods, and, of course, you can substitute those with another healthy food you like.

Yes, these are on my grocery list, but buy what is within *your* reach.

Everyday Food Portions/Substitutes

As I mentioned earlier, where I found myself in terms of food is portion control and substitutions, which I say to "eat everything but nothing". Are you wondering how? Let me explain.

- Do you know that breakfast is your most important meal of the day?
- Do you know you can eat five times a day and still maintain your desired shape/size by keeping your metabolism in balance?

A healthy metabolism needs many nutrients to function properly. In other words, the type of foods eaten can influence your metabolism. Food can be burned to provide energy, converted into body weight, or excreted.

Again, you don't want to feel like you are on a diet. You don't want to miss all your favourite meals and foods. Follow these steps and build your discipline based on portion control.

My best help to portion control includes the following.

- *Food prep:* Weekly meal prep is a good way to control meals as well as know your daily nutrient intake. Not that you are counting, but trust me: knowing your nutritional intake helps build your discipline.
- *Drink a glass of water before eating:* When I drink glass of water before eating, I literally don't feel the need to clear the whole plate. So I eat a little bit of it to satisfy the needs for taste and to chew.
- *Don't eat from bags or boxes:* You have no idea how many chips you consume when you eat from the bag, which is absolutely is not

necessary. When I buy a snack product that is supposed to have ten servings, I divide into ten bags or boxes ahead of time. That way I know exactly how much I have eaten.

- *Taste to be satisfied:* Trust me when I say Danish people have lots of sauces, and they all taste really good. I believe in the school of thought that one way to a man's heart is through his stomach, and I can't deny my man the foods he grew up with. Thus, I am a pro at making Danish *mormor* (grandma) sauces. But then I serve and take a little portion just for taste. I always tell myself I don't have drown my plate in the sauce to taste it, and it always work.

- *Keep the rest for tomorrow:* Oh, this is the part most of us fail. You made this delicious meal, and with the taste, you can finish a pot. When you have done all the above and still have the urge to keep eating because of the taste, just ask yourself: Is it necessary? And then remember you can have the rest tomorrow.

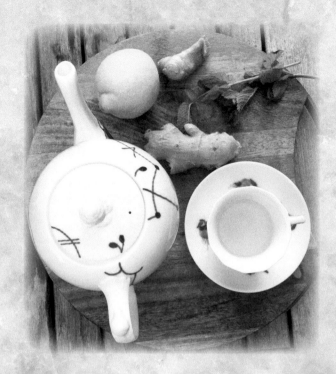

- *Sweet tooth treats:* For those who like to have something sweet after a meal, you don't have to miss it. You can swap for a new, healthier ritual as a signal that you're done eating. A good cup of tea with the desired flavour is always a good sweet tooth satisfier. (Homemade ginger tea flavoured with lemon, honey, and mint leaves is my preference.) But hey, I do have a bite of dark chocolate once in a while. It won't hurt.

Let me give you example of foods that you can substitute for others.

- brown rice or quinoa for white rice
- whole wheat bread or banana bread for white bread
- avocado puree instead of butter on bread
- mustard for mayonnaise

Food Ideas

Breakfast

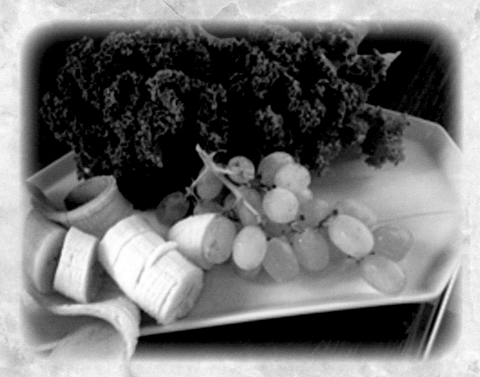

- smoothies made with kale, bananas, and green grapes

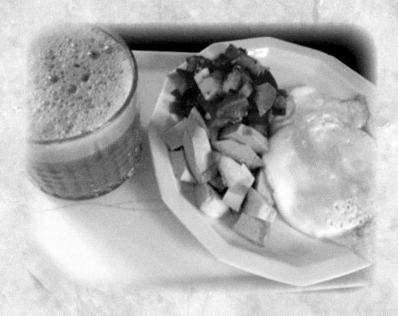

- pan-fried egg
- avocado
- tomato slices sprinkled with salt and pepper

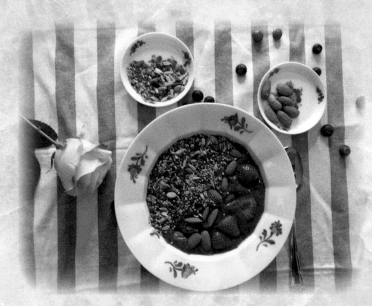

Lunch

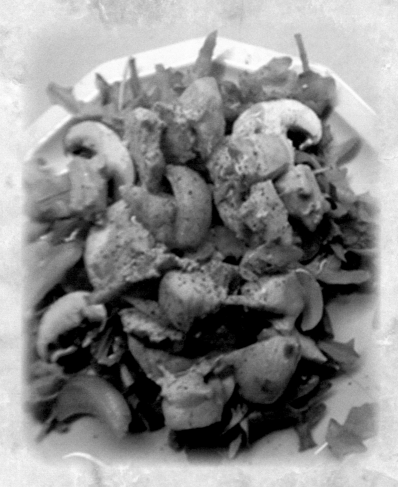

- lettuce or other green salad leaves
- tomato, sliced
- mushroom, sliced
- onion

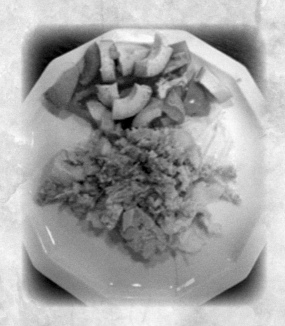

- pan-fried chicken breast
- avocado
- tuna

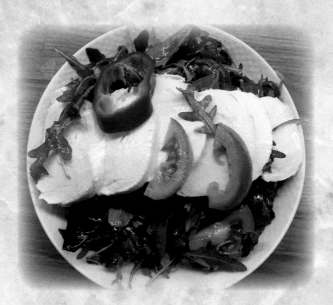

Dinner

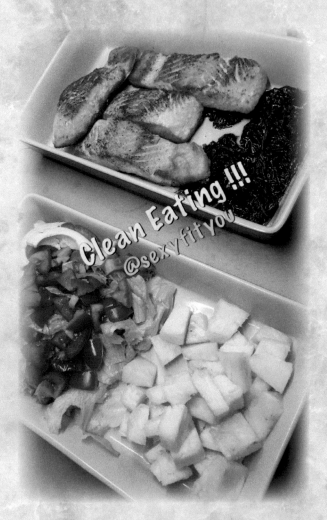

Clean Eating !!!
@sexyfityou

- salmon
- spinach
- pineapple
- tomato
- cabbage

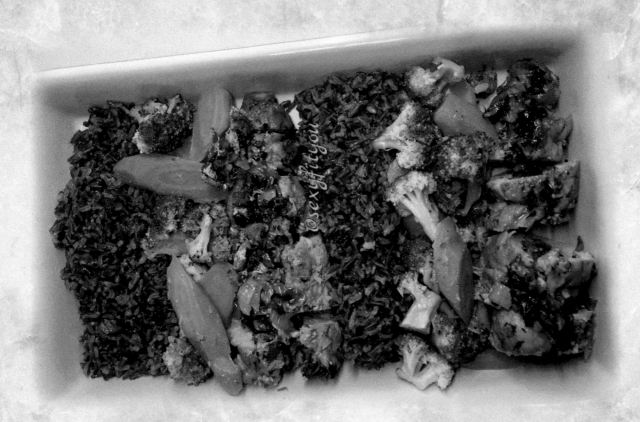

- brown rice
- broccoli
- carrot
- pork
- mushrooms
- chili pepper
- salt
- olive oil
- onions
- persil leaves

Note: Stuff pork with mushroom slices, chili pepper, parsley leaves, and onions. Sprinkle with salt and black pepper for flavour. Preheat oven at 180 degrees, put in your prep meal for forty-five minutes.

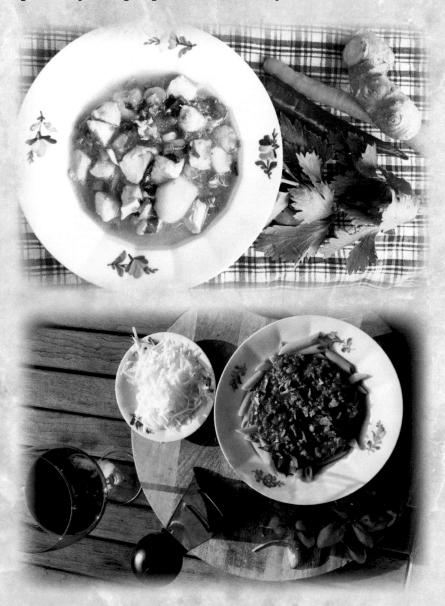

Basic Home Exercises

Description Box

Knee crunches , Bend your knees , then lift your left knee toward your right elbow ,lie back again, and your right knee towards your left elbow, allow your shoulder to do the elbow movement and you should be able to feel it in your tummy.

Cross fit crunches , Lie flat on your back and place your hands behind your head and then you tighten up your abs. You then lift your head and shoulders upwards but try not come all the way up off the floor like you do with a sit up.

Both side crunches lie flat on your back and straight out your hands by your sides , lean upwards and fold your knee , slide your hand and finger to touch the heel of your feet .

Squats simply describe as sit on the air , then stand straight again and tighten the boot

Reps points at how many times to count when performing the exercise whereas X points at how many time each rep is repeated

Abs:

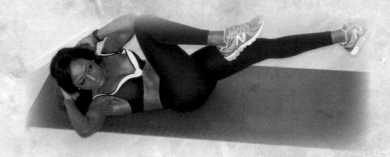

- knee crunches   15 reps x 3
- cross-feet crunches   15 reps x 3
- both-side crunches   10 reps x 2
- sixty second plank

Booty:

- prisoner squats   20 reps x 3
- jump squats   20 reps x 2
- waist lift butt crunch   10 reps x 3

Toned legs and thighs:

- wall sit   1 min x 3
- lunges   15 reps x 3
- front kicks   10 reps x 3
- rope skipping   20 reps x 3

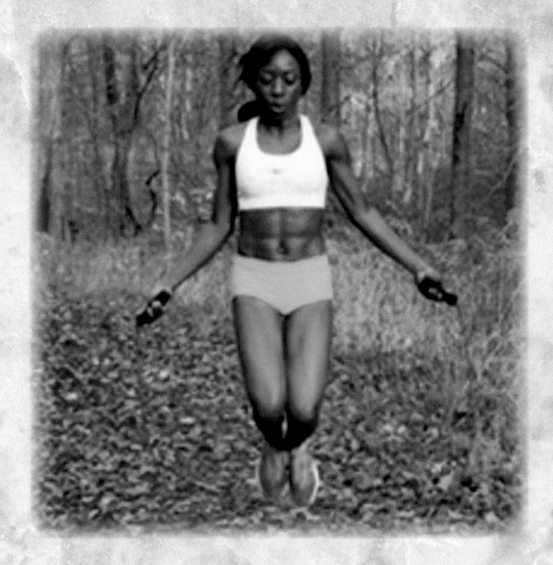

My seven-minute to-go exercises, which can literally be done with no clothes on while brushing your teeth in the morning, at your workplace, and so on, follow.

- Squats: First, while I brush my teeth, I do twenty squats and ten back kicks {kick your legs backwards in upward position} on both legs.

Second, I will ask you how many times do you pee in a day? That's how many times you should squat in a day. Simply do ten squats at each pee break. If you pee ten times in a day, that's one hundred squats you have kicked in.

- Knee Crunches: Before I take my shower after kicking in squats while brushing my teeth, I put my towel on the bathroom floor, lie back (probably on bare butt), and I knee crunches, counting to one hundred. Start with ten and increase with time.

Post-Partum

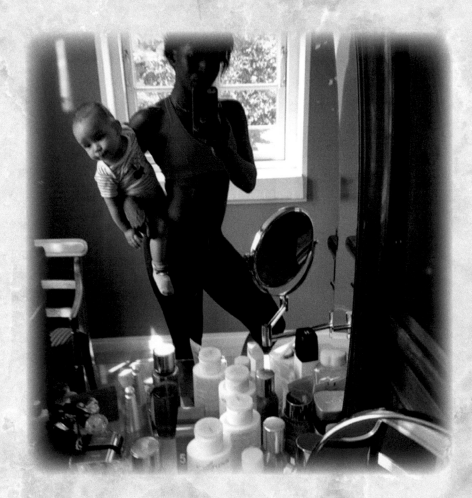

This is as real as it gets with me. I would have, of course, taken a professional picture with tummy all sucked in in order to prove something, but no. I choose to share with you this random unplanned, unprepared picture. Yet the picture says it all. Our daughter was precisely eight months when this picture was taken.

Telling you it's easy would also be lying to myself. It wasn't easy. But it's worth doing and trust me: your energy level doubles up.

Yes, recently post-partum is every woman's nightmare. With the challenges on social media these days, most women are just thinking and worrying of how to #snapback after giving birth, the ultimate worry of most mothers-to-be—even those yet to conceive. Maybe you're expecting me to say that I didn't have the same worry. Oh no! I was worried but in a different way. When I was told I couldn't have a normal delivery because of placenta position, first, I was sad that I wouldn't experience vaginal delivery. Then came the second worry/questioning: How long would it take before I could start exercising?

Although, deep down, I reminded myself of the discipline I had built and I knew I could maintain being SexyFit. I did, and so can you.

Let get you started.

- It all starts long before you conceive.
- First enjoy being a mother, take your time but keep the alarm at the back of your head.
- Stay on your portion control. As breastfeeding mothers, some of us think that we are eating for two, blah blah blah. Of course, consult with your doctor for your personal needs.
- Consult with your doctor as to when you should start exercising, but meanwhile, rocking your baby in the baby stroller for long-distance work is a great start.
- Bear in mind that every woman's body and the circumstances before, during, and after given birth are different.

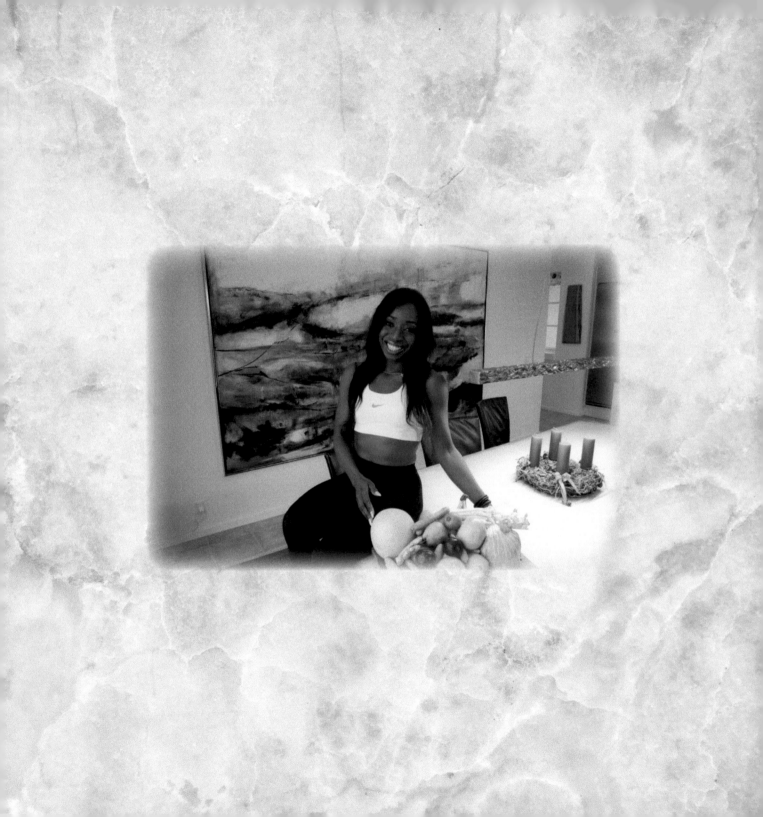

Author Description

Clara Chizoba Kronborg is a Nigerian-born, Denmark-based entrepreneur, media producer, presenter, event compere, and certified fitness coach. All her work, thus far, revolves around inspiring, motivating, and elevating women, hence the purpose of writing her first-ever book, *SexyFitYou*.

Clara's quest for a healthy lifestyle has existed since she was a teenager, but she has for the past eight years focused on building her understanding of her own body and its needs, even after giving birth.

About the Book

SexyFitYou is written by a woman for women. Not a conventional fitness book, there is absolutely zero dieting required. It is straight on building a positive lifestyle and self-love.

I dedicate this book to my mother, who was true to herself. She worked so hard all her life to impact and preserve a hardworking, family-oriented mindset within the family and the women around her. She was a woman who shared the little that she had with widows and women in difficulties. My desire to elevate, inspire, and motivate obviously comes from her, and I am privileged and humbled to share this journey with you.

Acknowledgements

Thank you to my husband, who has supported me in so many ways in making this dream a reality; to my daughter, in whose innocent eyes, I get more inspired each day; to my family and friends, who have stood by me, come rain, come shine; and to my publishers for a job well done.

Printed in the United States
By Bookmasters